HACK THAT GL

Balance Your Blood Sugar, Eat What You Need

Dr. Ruby J. James

DISCLAIMER

TABLE OF CONTENTS

INTRODUCTION: THE GLUCOSE IMPACT

Oh, sugar, sugar! It's not only a retro song from the '60s; it's also a tiny molecule that has a significant impact on the composition of your body's symphony of health. Welcome to the world of blood sugar, where your health can be made or destroyed by the enchanted glucose molecule's mystical ups and downs. So fasten your seatbelts as we explore the effects of blood sugar on your health!

From Highs to Lows on the Glucose Roller Coaster

Imagine your blood sugar skyrocketing when you down a sugary soda, like on a roller coaster. You get an energy rush, but alas, everything that rises must inevitably descend.

You find yourself in a slump and needing another sweet fix when your blood sugar levels fall. The cycle of highs and lows that can mess with your emotions, energy, and focus starts at this point.

Hungry Monsters Come Together!

Oh, those monsters of rage that appear as your blood sugar plummets! We've all been there: rumbling tummies, irritable disposition, ready to eat everybody in our path. Low blood sugar makes us vicious monsters until we satiate our needs, similar to an invitation to a angry party.

When Glucose Meets Sleep

Ever felt like a zombie getting by the day on little sleep? Guess what, though? This late-night drama also has blood sugar as a leading character!

When all you want is a peaceful night's sleep, unbalanced blood sugar levels conflict with your sleep patterns and cause you toss and turn.

The Acne-Aging Duo

Oh, the tempting sweets! While indulging in those sugary goodies may satisfy your palate, they might harm your skin as well! Spikes in blood sugar set off a hormonal dance that causes acne outbreaks and hastens the aging process. Who knew that glucose regulation held the key to eternal youth?

Taming the Hormones

Do your hormones ever seem to have a mind of their own, ladies? The blood sugar roller coaster is to blame. Your hormones are severely harmed by unstable glucose levels, which can lead to mood swings, PMS symptoms, and irregular cycles. But don't worry—we know how to tame the hormone dragon!

Glucose and Chronic Diseases

Watch out, since the hidden extra sugar in your system could lead to a variety of chronic illnesses! Uncontrolled blood sugar levels can have serious repercussions, ranging from the ominous specter of type 2 diabetes to heart disease and even dementia. But don't worry—we'll show you who the concealed evil is by revealing the hero!

Sweet Science Saves the Day!
Do not be alarmed, my friend, for it is possible to learn the beautiful science of blood sugar management! To regulate your blood sugar levels and open the doors to greater health, we provide you the science-backed secret elixir of easy hacks. Leaving the blood sugar roller coaster behind and welcoming a harmonic symphony of life!

It's time to go out on a pleasant tour through the realm of blood sugar and its wacky effects on your health, dear explorers. You will triumph over the sweet symphony of life armed with knowledge and tricks, dancing to the beat of wellbeing and happiness! Are you prepared to embark on this sugary adventure? Let's move!

The Effectiveness of Science-Based Techniques for Changing Blood Sugar

Ah, the science's magic! Science-based tips can transform your health journey into an engrossing story of energy and balance when it comes to the mysterious world of blood sugar.

As we reveal the incredible power of these techniques and their effect on your blood sugar metamorphosis, get ready to be mesmerized.

When it comes to blood sugar, have you ever felt as though you are trying to comprehend a mysterious code? Do not be alarmed; scientific hacks are here to solve the mystery!

These tips go deeply into the complex mechanisms of glucose regulation, giving you new perspectives on how your body regulates carbohydrates and how to keep that elusive balance.

Accurately Tapping into Your Cravings

Cravings are sneaky saboteurs that whisper tempting temptations in your ear. But using scientific tricks, you'll be able to trick those desires! With the help of these tricks, you may retrain your brain's pleasure centers to make you seek healthy meals while indulging in less reckless, more mindful ways.

Energizing Breakfasts to Power Your Day

According to science-based hacks, breakfast is the most crucial meal of the day. Learn how to make stimulating breakfasts that will keep your blood sugar stable and your energy levels high. Bid adieu to mid-morning slumps and welcome a day filled with vigor.

The Dessert Conundrum Is Overcome

Who says sweets and blood sugar can't live in peace with one another? The secret element to enjoying your favorite sweets while controlling your blood sugar is revealed via science-based hacks. Say goodbye to indulgences that make you feel bad and hello to pleasure that makes you feel good!

The Fountain of Youth and Glucose

The eternal attempt to halt aging's unrelenting advance. Here come the defenders of the fountain of youth: science-based hacks! These tips demonstrate how controlling your blood sugar can delay the onset of aging, preserving youthful skin, vivacious energy, and general wellbeing.

A Defense against Chronic Illnesses

Science-based hacks are your impenetrable defense in the war against chronic illnesses! Uncontrolled blood sugar can lead to a variety of health problems, but using these tips will strengthen your defenses and lower your risk of developing disorders like type 2 diabetes, heart disease, and other problems.

Empowerment and Better Health

At the core of science-based hacks is empowerment—the ability to reshape your life and take charge of your health.

Knowing and comprehending will enable you to make wise decisions, adopt a balanced lifestyle, and enjoy the sweetness of wellbeing.

To sum up, the effectiveness of scientifically proven techniques for lowering blood sugar is nothing short of amazing. These strategies are the key to learning how to manage your blood sugar, opening the door to a healthier, more energetic you.

So, go off on this fascinating transformational trip, guided by the wonders of science, and savor the sweet symphony of stable blood sugar levels and excellent health!

Chapter ONE: BUSTING THE GLUCOSE MYTH

Blood sugar management, the enigmatic dance of glucose in our bodies, frequently causes confusion and misunderstanding. It's time to bust myths and uncover facts regarding this critical part of our health. Let's cut through the misinformation and shine a light on the realities of blood sugar management.

Only for Diabetics

Oh, the age-old misconception! Blood sugar control is important for everyone's health, not only diabetics. Maintaining balanced blood sugar levels influences your energy, mood, skin, and overall health, whether you're a sugar addict or a health-conscious individual. It is a global search for energy!

No Carbs Allowed

Carbohydrates are frequently portrayed as villains in the blood sugar tale, causing some to feel that completely avoiding them is the solution. But wait a minute! Carbohydrates are not all made equal. It's not about eliminating carbs totally, but about making wise choices.

Abandon processed and sugary foods in favor of nutritious grains, fruits, and vegetables. Balance is essential!

Substitute Sweeteners

Many people feel that substituting artificial sweeteners or sugar replacements for sugar is the ultimate method for guilt-free enjoyment. Unfortunately, it is not that simple! While these choices are lower in calories, they can still have an influence on blood sugar and pose other health hazards. Natural sweeteners and moderation are better options.

Snacking is Bad

To snack or not to nibble: that is the question. Snacking isn't always bad in and of itself, but mindless snacking on sugary snacks can wreak havoc on blood sugar levels. Instead, choose healthy snacks that contain fiber, protein, and healthy fats to keep you content and your blood sugar stable.

Sugar Spikes Mean Trouble

Blood sugar spikes aren't necessarily the bad guys they're painted to be. It's normal for blood sugar levels to rise after a meal. The important factor is how rapidly it rises and how effectively your body handles it. Gradual and controlled spikes are preferable to abrupt surges.

Supplements Fix All

While vitamins can be beneficial, they cannot fix blood sugar problems on their own. They perform best when combined with a healthy diet and lifestyle.

Rather than relying entirely on supplements, concentrate on making long-term adjustments to your whole health regimen.

It's All About Diet

Blood sugar control isn't only about what you eat. Yes, diet is important, but other factors such as exercise, stress management, sleep, and overall lifestyle all have an impact on your glucose levels. Addressing the entire picture ensures complete blood sugar balance.

It's the All-in-One solution

Everybody is different, and blood sugar regulation is no exception. What works for one person might not work for another. Personalization is essential! Experiment with various tactics and watch how your body reacts. It's an exciting journey.

Chapter TWO: WHY THE HACK?

Consider this: you wake up feeling revitalized, ready to face the day with abundant energy. Your body vibrates with energy, and every work feels effortless. How do you get this wondrous condition of being? The answer is to master the art of glucose regulation, which is a powerful key to increasing energy efficiency and vigor.

The Glucose-Energy Relationship

Glucose, the tiny molecule with a big punch! Glucose, as the principal source of energy for our cells, is critical in powering our daily activities. However, in order to effectively harness its power, we must maintain a delicate balance.

Blood sugar fluctuations can cause energy surges and dumps, leaving us exhausted and fatigued.

Consistent Fuel for Maximum Performance

Consider your body to be a highly tuned machine that requires the correct fuel to work optimally. Blood sugar balance provides the consistent fuel required for peak performance.

A well-managed glucose system keeps you energized and focused, whether you're tackling professional chores, exercising, or simply spending time with loved ones.

Getting Rid of Brain Fog

Have you ever felt like your head is enveloped in a cloud of fog, making it difficult to concentrate? It's all due to shifting blood sugar levels!

Managing our glucose levels not only fuels our muscles but also feeds our brains. Stable blood sugar promotes mental clarity, keen focus, and increased cognitive function, allowing us to navigate the day with ease.

The Energy-Sleep Nexus

The interaction between glucose management and sleep quality is a delicate ballet. Uncontrolled blood sugar levels can alter sleep patterns, resulting in sleepless evenings and foggy mornings. Balanced glucose levels, on the other hand, promote better sleep, boosting the body's renewal process and ensuring you wake up ready to face the day.

The Endurance Sustainer

Glucose management is a game changer for fitness enthusiasts and sportsmen! Using glucose efficiently during exercise increases endurance and helps minimize weariness. Maintaining a healthy blood sugar profile throughout physical activity guarantees that you have the endurance to go the distance.

The Energy Ecosystem

Consider glucose control to be an orchestra conductor, balancing your body's whole energy environment. When your blood sugar is balanced, your hormones, metabolism, and total energy production all work together to create a symphony of vitality and well-being.

Chapter THREE: THE GLUCOSE HACK!

Blood sugar regulation does not have to be a difficult riddle to solve. In truth, there are very simple and efficient methods for keeping your glucose levels stable and dancing to a harmonious melody. Let's take a look at some basic techniques that can make a big difference in your blood sugar journey:

The Eating Method

Begin your day with a nutritious breakfast and build a meal schedule. Avoid missing meals or going too long without eating, as this can result in blood sugar swings. Mindful eating allows you to taste your food, control portion sizes, and keep your glucose levels stable throughout the day.

The Fiber-Rich Buddies

Fiber is the unsung blood sugar management hero! To delay the absorption of sugar into the bloodstream, include whole grains, fruits, vegetables, and legumes in your diet. The steady release of glucose aids in preventing those unexpected surges and crashes.

Smart Carbohydrates

Carbohydrates are not the enemy; it is all about choosing the appropriate ones! Choose complex carbs such as sweet potatoes, quinoa, and brown rice over refined and sugary carbohydrates.

These complex carbohydrates give a consistent supply of energy, keeping your blood sugar stable.

Protein Power

Including protein in your meals helps to keep blood sugar levels stable. Protein slows carbohydrate digestion, preventing fast surges. Include lean meats, fish, eggs, tofu, and beans to round up your protein intake.

Get Moving

Exercise is more than simply a calorie burner; it also regulates blood sugar levels! Physical activity improves insulin sensitivity, allowing your body to better utilize glucose. Even a short walk after meals will help keep blood sugar levels in balance.

Stay Hydrated

Water is the elixir of life, and it also helps to regulate blood sugar levels. Dehydration can result in elevated blood sugar levels, so drink lots of water throughout the day.

Avoid Sugary Drinks

Sugary beverages, such as sodas and fruit juices, might have a negative impact on your blood sugar levels. For a refreshing and blood sugar-friendly option, choose water, herbal teas, or sparkling water with a splash of citrus.

Stress Down!

Stress and blood sugar are inextricably linked in their own dance. Blood sugar abnormalities can result from chronic stress. To keep stress at bay and your glucose in balance, try relaxing techniques like meditation, yoga, or deep breathing.

Just Sleep!

Quality sleep is a secret weapon for blood sugar regulation. Sleep deprivation can affect hormones that regulate blood sugar, resulting in imbalances.

To improve your general health, aim for 7-9 hours of restful sleep per night.

Monitor and Learn

Monitor your blood sugar levels closely, especially if you have any pre-existing diseases. Keep track of how your body reacts to different diets and lifestyle changes. Understanding your body's unique sensitivities can allow you to fine-tune your blood sugar management.

Distraction Power

When cravings hit you hard, distraction might be your best friend. Engaging in an enjoyable hobby, going for a stroll, or spending time with loved ones might divert your attention away from the tempting treats. Cravings will soon lose their hold on your mind.

A Success Plan

Preparation is essential for defeating urges. Stock your pantry and refrigerator with healthy, filling snacks. Having healthy options on hand minimizes the likelihood of falling to less nutritious options.

Move On from Mistakes

Occasional indulgence is a part of life, and it's important to enjoy it guilt-free. Don't berate yourself if you give in to a craving. Instead, forgive yourself and renew your commitment to your journey of mindful eating and blood sugar balancing.

Controlling your cravings and curbing sweet temptations requires recognizing the triggers, employing clever tactics, and developing a healthy relationship with food. We unleash the power to resist cravings and restore control of our well-being by mastering the art of mindful eating, researching better choices, and nourishing our bodies with balanced meals. So, let us go on this journey of empowerment and submit to our newfound strength!

Chapter FOUR: THE AGEING HACK!

Aging is the eternal dance of time and our bodies. While we can't stop the clock, we can use a powerful tool to mitigate its effects: glucose management. Yes, you read that correctly! Managing glucose isn't just about energy and health; it also contains the secret to unlocking the fountain of youth. Let's look at some age-defying methods that highlight the enthralling link between glucose management and elegant aging.

The Sweet Science of Aging

To grasp the age-defying miracle of glucose regulation, we must first understand aging science. Oxidative stress, which causes cell damage and inflammation, is one of the fundamental causes of aging. Guess what can contribute to oxidative stress. You guessed it—uncontrolled glucose levels! Managing glucose effectively lowers oxidative stress, which aids in the preservation of youthful vitality.

The Glucose-Skin Relationship

The skin, our radiant armor, bears the brunt of the effects of aging. Wrinkles, fine lines, and elasticity loss—aging appears unstoppable.

Balanced blood sugar levels, on the other hand, have the potential to protect the skin from premature aging.

Elevated blood sugar causes glycation, a process that affects collagen and elastin, the building blocks of youthful skin. Glycation is controlled by glucose management, retaining skin suppleness and brightness.

Youth Powerhouses

The mitochondria, or powerhouses of energy generation, are found deep within our cells. As we age, mitochondrial activity might deteriorate, resulting in weariness and diminished vigor. But don't worry! Effective glucose management efficiently fuels the mitochondria, giving life to your energy factories and leaving you feeling youthful and bright.

Inflammation Tamer

Inflammation, the silent saboteur, is important in aging. Uncontrolled inflammation contributes to a number of age-related diseases. Blood sugar balance functions as a soft salve, easing inflammation and promoting general wellness.

By controlling inflammation, glucose management becomes a formidable barrier against premature aging.

The Ageless Diet and the Glycemic Index

The glycemic index (GI) contains the key to a youthful diet. Foods with a high GI cause fast spikes in blood sugar, which can accelerate the aging process.

By eating low-GI foods like whole grains, legumes, and veggies, you are embracing a healthy diet that maintains glucose levels and promotes youthful vitality.

Cognitive Clarity

Aging gracefully includes mental acuity as well. Managing glucose improves cognitive function, avoiding age-related cognitive decline and improving memory. You'll be able to navigate the years with a clear, agile mind if your blood sugar is balanced.

A Balanced Approach to life Age-defying hacks are more than simply short solutions; they represent a holistic approach to life. Adopt a healthy lifestyle that includes mindful eating, frequent exercise, stress management, and adequate rest.

A symbiotic dance of these factors, powered by glucose regulation, lays the groundwork for elegant aging.

Chapter FIVE: THE HORMONAL HACK!

Hormones are the invisible maestros of our bodies, conducting a symphony of functions that govern our health. Hormonal imbalances, on the other hand, might cause a discordant tune, wreaking havoc on our health. Not to worry, we have the power to achieve hormonal balance through science-backed hacks. Let's look into these game-changing methods for balancing our hormones and paving the way for better health.

Deciphering the Hormonal Maze

Understanding the maze of hormonal balance is the first step toward obtaining balance. Each hormone is important, from thyroid hormones that govern metabolism to sex hormones that influence fertility and mood. Identifying the underlying causes of hormone abnormalities allows us to deploy targeted interventions.

The Glucose-Hormone Relationship

Surprisingly, glucose control and hormone balance work hand in hand. Blood sugar fluctuations can affect insulin levels, causing abnormalities in other hormones.

We produce a ripple effect of hormonal balance throughout the body by mastering glucose regulation.

Endorphins and Exercise

Engage in regular physical activity to release endorphins, which are powerful hormones! These natural mood boosters boost your mood, lower stress hormones like cortisol, and improve hormonal balance. A fun fitness program lays the groundwork for hormonal bliss.

Accept Healthy Fats

Healthy fats are essential for hormonal health! Consume avocados, nuts, seeds, and fatty fish as part of your diet. These fats serve as the building blocks for hormone manufacturing, ensuring that your hormonal ensemble is in perfect balance.

The Stress-Relieving Technique

Stress, a subtle disruptor of hormone homeostasis, necessitates a planned strategy. To reduce stress hormones and encourage peace into your life, try relaxation practices such as meditation, deep breathing, or yoga.

Hormones and Rest: Beauty Sleep

Sleep is the ultimate hormonal balancer! Make excellent sleep a priority to help with hormone control. Hormones such as growth hormone and melatonin work their magic during deep sleep, encouraging regeneration and overall well-being.

Mindful Eating for Hormonal Health

The practice of sustaining your body and soul, mindful eating, takes center stage. Select foods high in vitamins and minerals to help with hormone synthesis and balance. Include fiber to help digestion and hormone excretion, creating a hormonal refuge on your plate.

Look for Hormonal Health Allies

On this journey, medical specialists that specialize in hormonal health can be your advocates. They can assist you in identifying specific imbalances and directing you to specialized methods to attain hormonal balance.

Chapter SIX: THE DESERT HACK!

Desserts, the sweet ending to a meal, captivate our taste receptors and envelop us in a sugary embrace. However, guilt frequently follows us, reminding us of excesses that may not be in line with our health goals. But don't worry, with a few science-backed tricks, you can enjoy the sweet art of dessert guilt-free. Let's dive into these scrumptious tricks that will allow us to enjoy our favorite foods guilt-free.

Recognize the Value of Moderation

Moderation is the first rule of the beautiful art! Desserts can be a component of a healthy diet if consumed in moderation. Savoring a modest portion of your favorite pleasure allows you to enjoy without feeling guilty.

Magic of Balance and Pairing

Desserts combined with fiber-rich foods can work miracles! Fiber inhibits the absorption of sugar into the system, which prevents blood sugar rises. Add a handful of almonds, a sprinkle of chia seeds, or a dollop of Greek yogurt to your dessert for a guilt-free balance.

Fruitful Dreams

Fruits are nature's wonderful gift, full of flavor and nutrition. Incorporate fresh fruits into your sweets for natural sweetness and vitamin boosts. From berries to mangoes, the opportunities for guilt-free enjoyment are boundless.

Sugar Substitutes That Work

Replace refined sugar with healthier alternatives such as stevia, erythritol, or monk fruit sweetener. These sugar replacements give sweetness without generating quick blood sugar spikes, making them ideal baking partners. Sweet art can be used to provide nourishment as well as pleasure! Investigate recipes that have components high in healthful fats, fiber, and protein. Desserts can be a delicious way to get extra nutrition.

The Dark Chocolate Mysteries

Ah, dark chocolate—the dessert's dark knight! Dark chocolate, which is high in antioxidants and low in sugar, provides a guilt-free retreat into chocolaty heaven. To gain the health benefits, choose cultivars with a greater cocoa content.

Make Your Own Desserts

Make your own desserts to control the ingredients. Experiment with whole grain flours, natural sweeteners, and healthy fats to make guilt-free treats that fit your taste preferences and health goals.

Enjoy the Experience

Dessert isn't only about the taste—it's also about the experience! Slow down, mindfully taste each bite, and totally immerse yourself in the pleasure of the moment. When you love the experience, guilt fades away, leaving only pure pleasure.

Finally, the sweet art of dessert is a joyful trip in which science and pleasure intersect. By implementing these methods, we gain guilt-free indulgence, allowing us to enjoy the pleasures of desserts without jeopardizing our health. So, let us go on this delectable journey, experiencing every sweet moment to the utmost!

Printed in Great Britain
by Amazon

26665591R10020